This book is not intended as a substitute for the medical advice of a doctor. The reader should regularly consult a doctor in matters relating to their health, and especially with respect to any symptoms that may require a diagnosis or medical attention

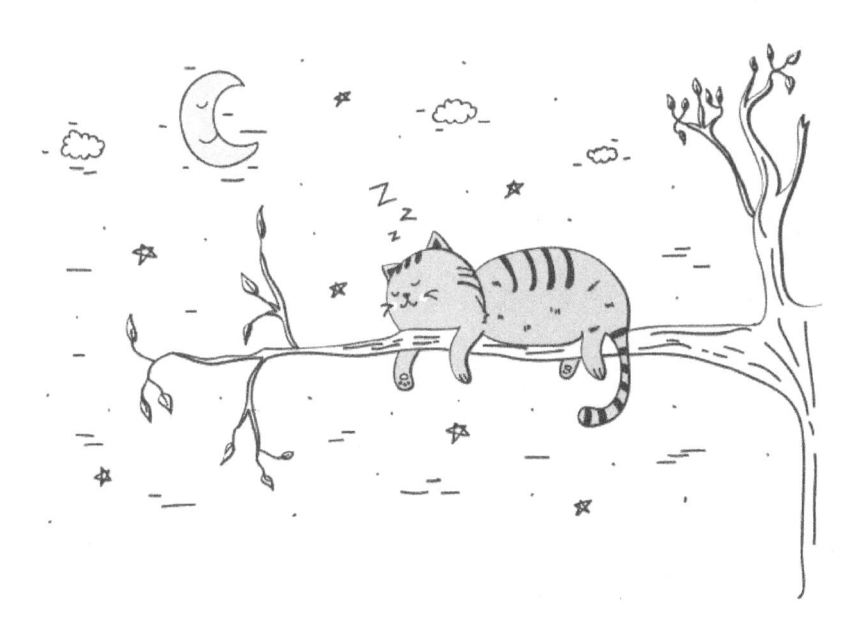

Art by Vecteezy.com; Text and design © 2019 by Duckie Journals

_____

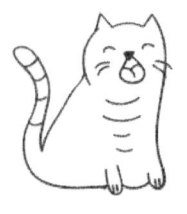

　　　　　Month　　　　　　*Year*

		1	2	3	4	5
6	7	8	9	10	11	12
13	14	15	16	17	18	19
20	21	22	23	24	25	26
27	28	29	30	31		

Days Since Last Period: ☐

Count the number of days in between the first day of each cycle, then take the average of several cycles to find out how long your cycles are!

Key
- ♦ Light
- ♦♦ Medium
- ♦♦♦ Heavy

Cramps? An over the counter medicine like ibuprofen (Motrin), naproxen (Aleve), or acetaminophen (Tylenol) can help! Make sure to check with your doctor first if you have any stomach or kidney problems

Record any symptoms you might have during your period, including cravings, your mood, cramps, aches, breast tenderness, and anything you did to feel better!

PMS Symptoms:

Day 1:

Day 2:

Day 3:

Day 4:

Day 5:

Day 6:

Day 7:

Notes:

_____ _____
Month   Year

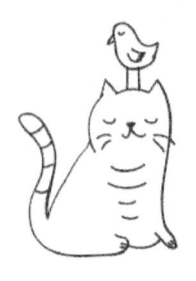

		1	2	3	4	5
6	7	8	9	10	11	12
13	14	15	16	17	18	19
20	21	22	23	24	25	26
27	28	29	30	31		

Days Since Last Period: ☐

Count the number of days in between the first day of each cycle, then take the average of several cycles to find out how long your cycles are!

Key

💧 Light
💧💧 Medium
💧💧💧 Heavy

Bloated? The sodium in salty foods can make bloating worse, so be sure to avoid any overly salty foods to help decrease water retention!

Record any symptoms you might have during your period, including cravings, your mood, cramps, aches, breast tenderness, and anything you did to feel better!

PMS Symptoms:

Day 1:

Day 2:

Day 3:

Day 4:

Day 5:

Day 6:

Day 7:

Notes:

Month   _Year_

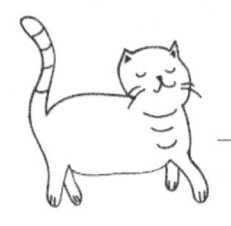

		1	2	3	4	5
6	7	8	9	10	11	12
13	14	15	16	17	18	19
20	21	22	23	24	25	26
27	28	29	30	31		

Days Since Last Period: ☐

Count the number of days in between the first day of each cycle, then take the average of several cycles to find out how long your cycles are!

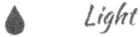

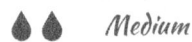

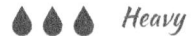

Key
- 💧 Light
- 💧💧 Medium
- 💧💧💧 Heavy

Bloated? Eating foods high in potassium may help reduce period bloating since potassium helps your body get rid of any excess sodium and water. Foods rich in potassium include spinach, bananas, avocados, and sweet potatoes

Record any symptoms you might have during your period, including cravings, your mood, cramps, aches, breast tenderness, and anything you did to feel better!

PMS Symptoms:

Day 1:

Day 2:

Day 3:

Day 4:

Day 5:

Day 6:

Day 7:

Notes:

_____ _____
              Month   Year

		1	2	3	4	5
6	7	8	9	10	11	12
13	14	15	16	17	18	19
20	21	22	23	24	25	26
27	28	29	30	31		

Days Since Last Period: ☐

Count the number of days in between the first day of each cycle, then take the average of several cycles to find out how long your cycles are!

Key

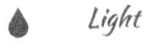

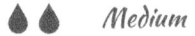

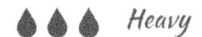

● Light
●● Medium
●●● Heavy

Cramps? A hot water bottle placed on the lower abdomen can help relieve the pain from period cramps. It's also great for backaches if placed on the back!

Record any symptoms you might have during your period, including cravings, your mood, cramps, aches, breast tenderness, and anything you did to feel better!

PMS Symptoms:

Day 1:

Day 2:

Day 3:

Day 4:

Day 5:

Day 6:

Day 7:

Notes:

Month   _Year_

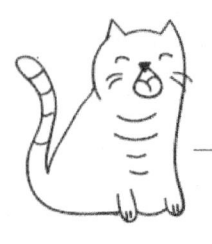

		1	2	3	4	5
6	7	8	9	10	11	12
13	14	15	16	17	18	19
20	21	22	23	24	25	26
27	28	29	30	31		

Days Since Last Period: ☐

Count the number of days in between the first day of each cycle, then take the average of several cycles to find out how long your cycles are!

Key

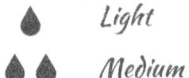

- ● Light
- ●● Medium
- ●●● Heavy

Bloated? Refined carbs such as white flour and processed sugars can cause your body to retain more sodium than usual, so try to avoid them if you can!

Record any symptoms you might have during your period, including cravings, your mood, cramps, aches, breast tenderness, and anything you did to feel better!

PMS Symptoms:

Day 1:

Day 2:

Day 3:

Day 4:

Day 5:

Day 6:

Day 7:

Notes:

_____
     Month   Year

		1	2	3	4	5
6	7	8	9	10	11	12
13	14	15	16	17	18	19
20	21	22	23	24	25	26
27	28	29	30	31		

Days Since Last Period: [　]

Count the number of days in between the first day of each cycle, then take the average of several cycles to find out how long your cycles are!

Key

- 💧 Light
- 💧💧 Medium
- 💧💧💧 Heavy

All that bleeding during your period can put you at risk for anemia. Be sure to eat plenty of foods rich in iron such as spinach, tuna, eggs, beef, tofu, and oysters.

Record any symptoms you might have during your period, including cravings, your mood, cramps, aches, breast tenderness, and anything you did to feel better!

PMS Symptoms:

Day 1:

Day 2:

Day 3:

Day 4:

Day 5:

Day 6:

Day 7:

Notes:

_____ _____
Month   Year

		1	2	3	4	5
6	7	8	9	10	11	12
13	14	15	16	17	18	19
20	21	22	23	24	25	26
27	28	29	30	31		

Days Since Last Period: ☐

Count the number of days in between the first day of each cycle, then take the average of several cycles to find out how long your cycles are!

Key
- ● Light
- ●● Medium
- ●●● Heavy

PMS? There's a reason for the chocolate cravings! Dark chocolate is rich in antioxidants which can reduce stress hormones. It also contains other substances that may enhance your mood. Just be sure to only go for dark chocolate that's at least 60% cacao.

Record any symptoms you might have during your period, including cravings, your mood, cramps, aches, breast tenderness, and anything you did to feel better!

PMS Symptoms:

Day 1:

Day 2:

Day 3:

Day 4:

Day 5:

Day 6:

Day 7:

Notes:

_____ _____
Month   Year

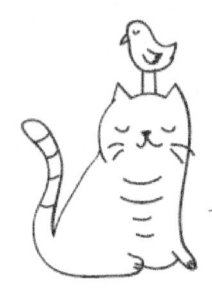

			1	2	3	4	5
6	7	8	9	10	11	12
13	14	15	16	17	18	19
20	21	22	23	24	25	26
27	28	29	30	31		

Days Since Last Period: ☐

Count the number of days in between the first day of each cycle, then take the average of several cycles to find out how long your cycles are!

Key
- 💧 Light
- 💧💧 Medium
- 💧💧💧 Heavy

Swollen breasts? Gently massaging your breasts can help the lymphatic system drain all that extra fluid out from them, easing the pain. Be sure to include your chest and armpit area in the massage, where a lot of lymph nodes are located!

Record any symptoms you might have during your period, including cravings, your mood, cramps, aches, breast tenderness, and anything you did to feel better!

PMS Symptoms:

Day 1:

Day 2:

Day 3:

Day 4:

Day 5:

Day 6:

Day 7:

Notes:

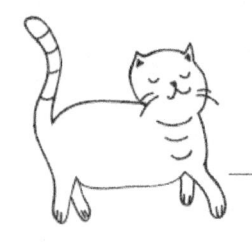

Month _Year_

		1	2	3	4	5
6	7	8	9	10	11	12
13	14	15	16	17	18	19
20	21	22	23	24	25	26
27	28	29	30	31		

Days Since Last Period:

Count the number of days in between the first day of each cycle, then take the average of several cycles to find out how long your cycles are!

Key

- 💧 Light
- 💧💧 Medium
- 💧💧💧 Heavy

PMS? Research suggests that omega-3 fatty acids can help reduce PMS symptoms. Foods rich in omega-3 fatty acids include mackerel, salmon, oysters, sardines, seaweed, chia seeds, and flaxseeds.

Record any symptoms you might have during your period, including cravings, your mood, cramps, aches, breast tenderness, and anything you did to feel better!

PMS Symptoms:

Day 1:

Day 2:

Day 3:

Day 4:

Day 5:

Day 6:

Day 7:

Notes:

Month _Year_

		1	2	3	4	5
6	7	8	9	10	11	12
13	14	15	16	17	18	19
20	21	22	23	24	25	26
27	28	29	30	31		

Days Since Last Period:

Count the number of days in between the first day of each cycle, then take the average of several cycles to find out how long your cycles are!

Key
- ● Light
- ●● Medium
- ●●● Heavy

Exercising during your period can release lots of mood-boosting endorphins which can also help relieve cramps, bloating, and lower back pain. Aim for at least 30 minutes of exercise 2-3 times a week regularly, but don't push yourself too hard during your period.

Record any symptoms you might have during your period, including cravings, your mood, cramps, aches, breast tenderness, and anything you did to feel better!

PMS Symptoms:

Day 1:

Day 2:

Day 3:

Day 4:

Day 5:

Day 6:

Day 7:

Notes:

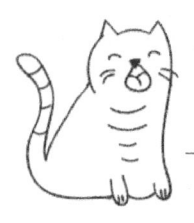

_____ _____
Month   Year

		1	2	3	4	5
6	7	8	9	10	11	12
13	14	15	16	17	18	19
20	21	22	23	24	25	26
27	28	29	30	31		

Days Since Last Period: ☐

Count the number of days in between the first day of each cycle, then take the average of several cycles to find out how long your cycles are!

Key
- ● Light
- ●● Medium
- ●●● Heavy

Yoga is great for helping with back pain. There are even many different poses to help with cramps! Some great yoga poses for menstrual pain include: the bound angle pose, the reclined bound angle pose, the child pose, and the reclining twist.

Record any symptoms you might have during your period, including cravings, your mood, cramps, aches, breast tenderness, and anything you did to feel better!

PMS Symptoms:

Day 1:

Day 2:

Day 3:

Day 4:

Day 5:

Day 6:

Day 7:

Notes:

_____
Month   Year

		1	2	3	4	5
6	7	8	9	10	11	12
13	14	15	16	17	18	19
20	21	22	23	24	25	26
27	28	29	30	31		

Days Since Last Period: ☐

Count the number of days in between the first day of each cycle, then take the average of several cycles to find out long your cycles are!

Key

- ♦ Light
- ♦♦ Medium
- ♦♦♦ Heavy

Laughing is a great way to ease stress and anxiety. Here's a joke to get you started: How do cats end a fight? They hiss and make up!

Record any symptoms you might have during your period, including cravings, your mood, cramps, aches, breast tenderness, and anything you did to feel better!

PMS Symptoms:

Day 1:

Day 2:

Day 3:

Day 4:

Day 5:

Day 6:

Day 7:

Notes:

Year End Summary:
Cycle Lengths

Month 1	
Month 2	
Month 3	
Month 4	
Month 5	
Month 6	
Month 7	
Month 8	
Month 9	
Month 10	
Month 11	
Month 12	

Average Cycle Length: _____

On to the next year!

_____
Month   Year

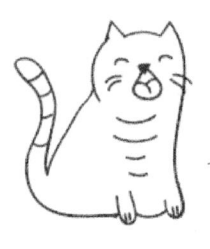

		1	2	3	4	5
6	7	8	9	10	11	12
13	14	15	16	17	18	19
20	21	22	23	24	25	26
27	28	29	30	31		

Days Since Last Period: ☐

Count the number of days in between the first day of each cycle, then take the average of several cycles to find out long your cycles are!

Key
- ● Light
- ●● Medium
- ●●● Heavy

Constipated? Some hormones released during certain times of the menstrual cycle can promote constipation. Remember to eat plenty of fiber regularly and stay hydrated.

Record any symptoms you might have during your period, including cravings, your mood, cramps, aches, breast tenderness, and anything you did to feel better!

PMS Symptoms:

Day 1:

Day 2:

Day 3:

Day 4:

Day 5:

Day 6:

Day 7:

Notes:

_____ _____
Month   Year

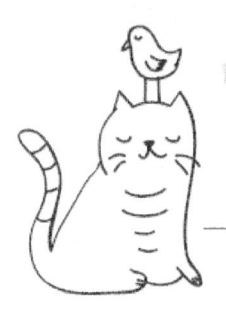

		1	2	3	4	5
6	7	8	9	10	11	12
13	14	15	16	17	18	19
20	21	22	23	24	25	26
27	28	29	30	31		

Days Since Last Period: ☐

Count the number of days in between the first day of each cycle, then take the average of several cycles to find out long your cycles are!

Key
- ● Light
- ●● Medium
- ●●● Heavy

Chemicals called prostaglandins are released when menstruation begins. They cause your intestines and uterus to contract, leading to diarrhea and cramps. Eating foods such as yogurt, sauerkraut, and kimchi can help keep your digestive system healthy since they contain beneficial bacteria such as lactobacillus.

Record any symptoms you might have during your period, including cravings, your mood, cramps, aches, breast tenderness, and anything you did to feel better!

PMS Symptoms:

Day 1:

Day 2:

Day 3:

Day 4:

Day 5:

Day 6:

Day 7:

Notes:

_____ _____
Month   Year

		1	2	3	4	5
6	7	8	9	10	11	12
13	14	15	16	17	18	19
20	21	22	23	24	25	26
27	28	29	30	31		

Days Since Last Period: ☐

Count the number of days in between the first day of each cycle, then take the average of several cycles to find out long your cycles are!

Key

- ● Light
- ●● Medium
- ●●● Heavy

Oral contraceptives are a great option for regulating periods. They can also help control heavy periods and decrease acne. Ask your doctor if they could be right for you.

Record any symptoms you might have during your period, including cravings, your mood, cramps, aches, breast tenderness, and anything you did to feel better!

PMS Symptoms:

Day 1:

Day 2:

Day 3:

Day 4:

Day 5:

Day 6:

Day 7:

Notes:

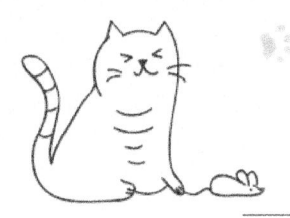

Month _____ Year _____

		1	2	3	4	5
6	7	8	9	10	11	12
13	14	15	16	17	18	19
20	21	22	23	24	25	26
27	28	29	30	31		

Days Since Last Period: ☐

Count the number of days in between the first day of each cycle, then take the average of several cycles to find out long your cycles are!

Key
- 💧 Light
- 💧💧 Medium
- 💧💧💧 Heavy

Cravings? Protein helps stabilize blood sugar and increase feelings of fullness after a meal. Including plenty of protein rich foods in your diet can help control cravings. High protein foods include eggs, nuts, dairy, seafood, and meat such as chicken breast.

Record any symptoms you might have during your period, including cravings, your mood, cramps, aches, breast tenderness, and anything you did to feel better!

PMS Symptoms:

Day 1:

Day 2:

Day 3:

Day 4:

Day 5:

Day 6:

Day 7:

Notes:

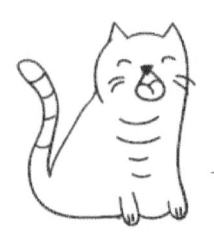

_____

Month   Year

		1	2	3	4	5
6	7	8	9	10	11	12
13	14	15	16	17	18	19
20	21	22	23	24	25	26
27	28	29	30	31		

Days Since Last Period: ☐

Count the number of days in between the first day of each cycle, then take the average of several cycles to find out long your cycles are!

Key
- ♦ Light
- ♦♦ Medium
- ♦♦♦ Heavy

PMS? Research has shown that women with higher intakes of calcium and vitamin D are less likely to develop PMS. Calcium from food is better absorbed than calcium from supplements. Calcium rich foods include milk, cheese, yogurt, and fortified orange juice or soymilk. Leafy greens are also a great source of calcium!

Record any symptoms you might have during your period, including cravings, your mood, cramps, aches, breast tenderness, and anything you did to feel better!

PMS Symptoms:

Day 1:

Day 2:

Day 3:

Day 4:

Day 5:

Day 6:

Day 7:

Notes:

_____ _____
Month   Year

		1	2	3	4	5
6	7	8	9	10	11	12
13	14	15	16	17	18	19
20	21	22	23	24	25	26
27	28	29	30	31		

Days Since Last Period: ☐

Count the number of days in between the first day of each cycle, then take the average of several cycles to find out long your cycles are!

Key

- 💧 Light
- 💧💧 Medium
- 💧💧💧 Heavy

Stress can contribute to how intense PMS symptoms are. Take a few minutes out of your day to relax and take a deep breath. There are also lots of great resources online on meditation.

Record any symptoms you might have during your period, including cravings, your mood, cramps, aches, breast tenderness, and anything you did to feel better!

PMS Symptoms:

Day 1:

Day 2:

Day 3:

Day 4:

Day 5:

Day 6:

Day 7:

Notes:

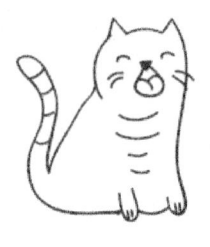

_____   _____
       Month   Year

		1	2	3	4	5
6	7	8	9	10	11	12
13	14	15	16	17	18	19
20	21	22	23	24	25	26
27	28	29	30	31		

Days Since Last Period: ☐

Count the number of days in between the first day of each cycle, then take the average of several cycles to find out long your cycles are!

Key

● Light
●● Medium
●●● Heavy

In addition to causing cancer and wrinkles, a recent study has shown that smoking, especially in early adulthood, may increase a woman's risk for PMS symptoms!

Record any symptoms you might have during your period, including cravings, your mood, cramps, aches, breast tenderness, and anything you did to feel better!

PMS Symptoms:

Day 1:

Day 2:

Day 3:

Day 4:

Day 5:

Day 6:

Day 7:

Notes:

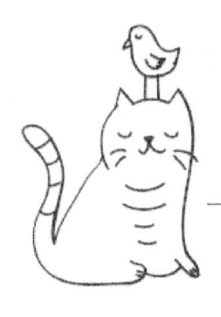

_____ _____
Month   Year

		1	2	3	4	5
6	7	8	9	10	11	12
13	14	15	16	17	18	19
20	21	22	23	24	25	26
27	28	29	30	31		

Days Since Last Period: ☐

Count the number of days in between the first day of each cycle, then take the average of several cycles to find out long your cycles are!

Key
- 💧 Light
- 💧💧 Medium
- 💧💧💧 Heavy

Bloated? It doesn't sound very intuitive, but drinking plenty of water can help with bloating. The water helps flush out extra sodium from your body, reducing water retention. How much water did you drink today?

Record any symptoms you might have during your period, including cravings, your mood, cramps, aches, breast tenderness, and anything you did to feel better!

PMS Symptoms:

Day 1:

Day 2:

Day 3:

Day 4:

Day 5:

Day 6:

Day 7:

Notes:

_____ _____
Month   Year

		1	2	3	4	5
6	7	8	9	10	11	12
13	14	15	16	17	18	19
20	21	22	23	24	25	26
27	28	29	30	31		

Days Since Last Period: ☐

Count the number of days in between the first day of each cycle, then take the average of several cycles to find out long your cycles are!

Key
- ● Light
- ●● Medium
- ●●● Heavy

Feeling fatigued? PMS can cause you to feel extra tired compared to usual. It is important to have an established sleeping schedule and sleep on time every night. Aim for around 7 to 8 hours of beauty sleep each day.

Record any symptoms you might have during your period, including cravings, your mood, cramps, aches, breast tenderness, and anything you did to feel better!

PMS Symptoms:

Day 1:

Day 2:

Day 3:

Day 4:

Day 5:

Day 6:

Day 7:

Notes:

_____ _____
Month   Year

		1	2	3	4	5
6	7	8	9	10	11	12
13	14	15	16	17	18	19
20	21	22	23	24	25	26
27	28	29	30	31		

Days Since Last Period: ☐

Count the number of days in between the first day of each cycle, then take the average of several cycles to find out long your cycles are!

Key
- ♦ Light
- ♦♦ Medium
- ♦♦♦ Heavy

Being on your period may make you feel gross. But remember, your vagina is like a self-cleaning oven. You do not need to put anything inside to clean it. This includes douches, which can lead to vaginal infections!

Record any symptoms you might have during your period, including cravings, your mood, cramps, aches, breast tenderness, and anything you did to feel better!

PMS Symptoms:

Day 1:

Day 2:

Day 3:

Day 4:

Day 5:

Day 6:

Day 7:

Notes:

_____ _____
Month   Year

		1	2	3	4	5
6	7	8	9	10	11	12
13	14	15	16	17	18	19
20	21	22	23	24	25	26
27	28	29	30	31		

Days Since Last Period: ☐

Count the number of days in between the first day of each cycle, then take the average of several cycles to find out long your cycles are!

Key
- ● Light
- ●● Medium
- ●●● Heavy

Menstrual stains on your clothes? Soaking the item of clothing in cold water immediately can keep the blood from setting into the fabric. Follow with laundry soap as usual. For stubborn stains, hydrogen peroxide can help. Just remember to spot test an inconspicuous area first.

Record any symptoms you might have during your period, including cravings, your mood, cramps, aches, breast tenderness, and anything you did to feel better!

PMS Symptoms:

Day 1:

Day 2:

Day 3:

Day 4:

Day 5:

Day 6:

Day 7:

Notes:

Month   _Year_

		1	2	3	4	5
6	7	8	9	10	11	12
13	14	15	16	17	18	19
20	21	22	23	24	25	26
27	28	29	30	31		

Days Since Last Period: ☐

Count the number of days in between the first day of each cycle, then take the average of several cycles to find out long your cycles are!

Key

- 💧 Light
- 💧💧 Medium
- 💧💧💧 Heavy

Cramps? A natural way to help alleviate menstrual cramp pain is self massage. Massaging your lower abdomen (gently!) can encourage blood flow and relax the tense muscles. While you're at it, massage your lower back to help with any back pain.

Record any symptoms you might have during your period, including cravings, your mood, cramps, aches, breast tenderness, and anything you did to feel better!

PMS Symptoms:

Day 1:

Day 2:

Day 3:

Day 4:

Day 5:

Day 6:

Day 7:

Notes:

Year End Summary:
Cycle Lengths

Month 1	
Month 2	
Month 3	
Month 4	
Month 5	
Month 6	
Month 7	
Month 8	
Month 9	
Month 10	
Month 11	
Month 12	

Average Cycle Length: _____

On to the next year!

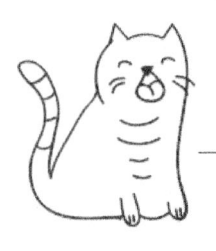

_____ _____
Month   Year

		1	2	3	4	5
6	7	8	9	10	11	12
13	14	15	16	17	18	19
20	21	22	23	24	25	26
27	28	29	30	31		

Days Since Last Period: ☐

Count the number of days in between the first day of each cycle, then take the average of several cycles to find out long your cycles are!

Key
- ● Light
- ●● Medium
- ●●● Heavy

Cramps? An over the counter medicine like ibuprofen (Motrin), naproxen (Aleve), or acetaminophen (Tylenol) can help! Make sure to check with your doctor first if you have any stomach or kidney problems.

Record any symptoms you might have during your period, including cravings, your mood, cramps, aches, breast tenderness, and anything you did to feel better!

PMS Symptoms:

Day 1:

Day 2:

Day 3:

Day 4:

Day 5:

Day 6:

Day 7:

Notes:

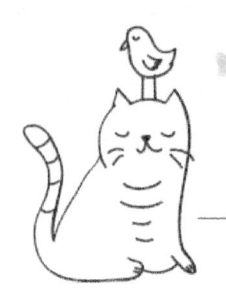

_____ _____
Month   Year

			1	2	3	4	5
6	7	8	9	10	11	12
13	14	15	16	17	18	19
20	21	22	23	24	25	26
27	28	29	30	31		

Days Since Last Period: ☐

Count the number of days in between the first day of each cycle, then take the average of several cycles to find out long your cycles are!

Key

- ● Light
- ●● Medium
- ●●● Heavy

Bloated? The sodium in salty foods can make bloating worse, so be sure to avoid any overly salty foods to help decrease water retention!

Record any symptoms you might have during your period, including cravings, your mood, cramps, aches, breast tenderness, and anything you did to feel better!

PMS Symptoms:

Day 1:

Day 2:

Day 3:

Day 4:

Day 5:

Day 6:

Day 7:

Notes:

_____ _____
Month   Year

		1	2	3	4	5
6	7	8	9	10	11	12
13	14	15	16	17	18	19
20	21	22	23	24	25	26
27	28	29	30	31		

Days Since Last Period: ☐

Count the number of days in between the first day of each cycle, then take the average of several cycles to find out long your cycles are!

Key
- ♦ Light
- ♦♦ Medium
- ♦♦♦ Heavy

Bloated? Eating foods high in potassium may help reduce period bloating since potassium helps your body get rid of any excess sodium and water. Foods rich in potassium include spinach, bananas, avocados, and sweet potatoes.

Record any symptoms you might have during your period, including cravings, your mood, cramps, aches, breast tenderness, and anything you did to feel better!

PMS Symptoms:

Day 1:

Day 2:

Day 3:

Day 4:

Day 5:

Day 6:

Day 7:

Notes:

_____
Month   Year

		1	2	3	4	5
6	7	8	9	10	11	12
13	14	15	16	17	18	19
20	21	22	23	24	25	26
27	28	29	30	31		

Days Since Last Period:

Count the number of days in between the first day of each cycle, then take the average of several cycles to find out long your cycles are!

Key

● Light
●● Medium
●●● Heavy

Bloated? Refined carbs such as white flour and processed sugars can cause your body to retain more sodium than usual.

Record any symptoms you might have during your period, including cravings, your mood, cramps, aches, breast tenderness, and anything you did to feel better!

PMS Symptoms:

Day 1:

Day 2:

Day 3:

Day 4:

Day 5:

Day 6:

Day 7:

Notes:

Month _Year_

		1	2	3	4	5
6	7	8	9	10	11	12
13	14	15	16	17	18	19
20	21	22	23	24	25	26
27	28	29	30	31		

Days Since Last Period:

Count the number of days in between the first day of each cycle, then take the average of several cycles to find out long your cycles are!

Key

- ♦ Light
- ♦♦ Medium
- ♦♦♦ Heavy

Cramps? A hot water bottle placed on the lower abdomen can help relieve the pain from period cramps. It's also great for period backaches when placed on the lower back!

Record any symptoms you might have during your period, including cravings, your mood, cramps, aches, breast tenderness, and anything you did to feel better!

PMS Symptoms:

Day 1:

Day 2:

Day 3:

Day 4:

Day 5:

Day 6:

Day 7:

Notes:

_____
Month   Year

		1	2	3	4	5
6	7	8	9	10	11	12
13	14	15	16	17	18	19
20	21	22	23	24	25	26
27	28	29	30	31		

Days Since Last Period: ☐

Count the number of days in between the first day of each cycle, then take the average of several cycles to find out long your cycles are!

Key

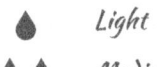

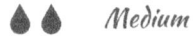

- 💧 Light
- 💧💧 Medium
- 💧💧💧 Heavy

All that bleeding during your period can put you at risk for anemia. Be sure to eat plenty of foods rich in iron such as spinach, tuna, eggs, beef, tofu, and oysters.

Record any symptoms you might have during your period, including cravings, your mood, cramps, aches, breast tenderness, and anything you did to feel better!

PMS Symptoms:

Day 1:

Day 2:

Day 3:

Day 4:

Day 5:

Day 6:

Day 7:

Notes:

_____ _____
Month   Year

		1	2	3	4	5
6	7	8	9	10	11	12
13	14	15	16	17	18	19
20	21	22	23	24	25	26
27	28	29	30	31		

Days Since Last Period: ☐

Count the number of days in between the first day of each cycle, then take the average of several cycles to find out long your cycles are!

Key
- ● Light
- ●● Medium
- ●●● Heavy

PMS? There's a reason for the chocolate cravings! Dark chocolate is rich in antioxidants which can reduce stress hormones and other substances that may enhance your mood. Just be sure to only go for dark chocolate that's at least 60% cacao.

Record any symptoms you might have during your period, including cravings, your mood, cramps, aches, breast tenderness, and anything you did to feel better!

PMS Symptoms:

Day 1:

Day 2:

Day 3:

Day 4:

Day 5:

Day 6:

Day 7:

Notes:

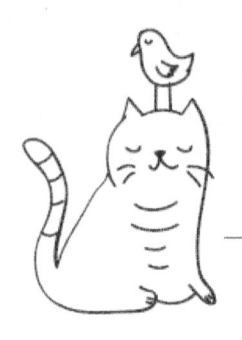

_____ Month _____ Year _____

		1	2	3	4	5
6	7	8	9	10	11	12
13	14	15	16	17	18	19
20	21	22	23	24	25	26
27	28	29	30	31		

Days Since Last Period: ☐

Count the number of days in between the first day of each cycle, then take the average of several cycles to find out long your cycles are!

Key

- 💧 Light
- 💧💧 Medium
- 💧💧💧 Heavy

Swollen breasts? Gently massaging your breasts can help the lymphatic system drain all that extra fluid out from them, easing the pain. Be sure to include your chest and armpit area, where a lot of lymph nodes are located!

Record any symptoms you might have during your period, including cravings, your mood, cramps, aches, breast tenderness, and anything you did to feel better!

PMS Symptoms:

Day 1:

Day 2:

Day 3:

Day 4:

Day 5:

Day 6:

Day 7:

Notes:

_____
Month   *Year*

		1	2	3	4	5
6	7	8	9	10	11	12
13	14	15	16	17	18	19
20	21	22	23	24	25	26
27	28	29	30	31		

Days Since Last Period: ☐

Count the number of days in between the first day of each cycle, then take the average of several cycles to find out long your cycles are!

Key
● *Light*
●● *Medium*
●●● *Heavy*

PMS? Research suggests that omega-3 fatty acids can help reduce PMS symptoms. Foods rich in omega-3s include mackerel, salmon, oysters, sardines, seaweed, chia seeds, and flaxseeds.

Record any symptoms you might have during your period, including cravings, your mood, cramps, aches, breast tenderness, and anything you did to feel better!

PMS Symptoms:

Day 1:

Day 2:

Day 3:

Day 4:

Day 5:

Day 6:

Day 7:

Notes:

_____ _____
Month   Year

		1	2	3	4	5
6	7	8	9	10	11	12
13	14	15	16	17	18	19
20	21	22	23	24	25	26
27	28	29	30	31		

Days Since Last Period: ☐

Count the number of days in between the first day of each cycle, then take the average of several cycles to find out long your cycles are!

Key

💧 Light
💧💧 Medium
💧💧💧 Heavy

Exercising during your period can release lots of mood-boosting endorphins which can also help with relieving cramps, bloating, and lower back pain.

Record any symptoms you might have during your period, including cravings, your mood, cramps, aches, breast tenderness, and anything you did to feel better!

PMS Symptoms:

Day 1:

Day 2:

Day 3:

Day 4:

Day 5:

Day 6:

Day 7:

Notes:

Month _Year_

		1	2	3	4	5
6	7	8	9	10	11	12
13	14	15	16	17	18	19
20	21	22	23	24	25	26
27	28	29	30	31		

Days Since Last Period:

Count the number of days in between the first day of each cycle, then take the average of several cycles to find out long your cycles are!

Key

● Light
●● Medium
●●● Heavy

Yoga is great for helping with back pain. There are even many different poses to help with cramps! Some great yoga poses include: the bound angle pose, reclined bound angle pose, the child pose, and the reclining twist.

Record any symptoms you might have during your period, including cravings, your mood, cramps, aches, breast tenderness, and anything you did to feel better!

PMS Symptoms:

Day 1:

Day 2:

Day 3:

Day 4:

Day 5:

Day 6:

Day 7:

Notes:

Month _Year_

		1	2	3	4	5
6	7	8	9	10	11	12
13	14	15	16	17	18	19
20	21	22	23	24	25	26
27	28	29	30	31		

Days Since Last Period:

Count the number of days in between the first day of each cycle, then take the average of several cycles to find out long your cycles are!

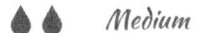

Key

- ● Light
- ●● Medium
- ●●● Heavy

Laughing is a great way to ease stress and anxiety. Here's a joke to get you started: What kind of cats go bowling?
Alley cats!

Record any symptoms you might have during your period, including cravings, your mood, cramps, aches, breast tenderness, and anything you did to feel better!

PMS Symptoms:

Day 1:

Day 2:

Day 3:

Day 4:

Day 5:

Day 6:

Day 7:

Notes:

Year End Summary:
Cycle Lengths

Month 1	
Month 2	
Month 3	
Month 4	
Month 5	
Month 6	
Month 7	
Month 8	
Month 9	
Month 10	
Month 11	
Month 12	

Average Cycle Length: _____

On to the next year!

_____
                Month   Year

		1	2	3	4	5
6	7	8	9	10	11	12
13	14	15	16	17	18	19
20	21	22	23	24	25	26
27	28	29	30	31		

Days Since Last Period: ☐

Count the number of days in between the first day of each cycle, then take the average of several cycles to find out long your cycles are!

Key

- ● Light
- ●● Medium
- ●●● Heavy

Constipated? Some of the hormones released during certain times of the menstrual cycle can promote constipation. Remember to eat plenty of fiber regularly and stay hydrated.

Record any symptoms you might have during your period, including cravings, your mood, cramps, aches, breast tenderness, and anything you did to feel better!

PMS Symptoms:

Day 1:

Day 2:

Day 3:

Day 4:

Day 5:

Day 6:

Day 7:

Notes:

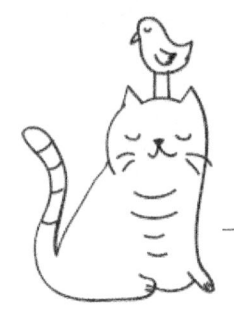

_____
     Month   Year

		1	2	3	4	5
6	7	8	9	10	11	12
13	14	15	16	17	18	19
20	21	22	23	24	25	26
27	28	29	30	31		

Days Since Last Period: ☐

Count the number of days in between the first day of each cycle, then take the average of several cycles to find out long your cycles are!

Key
- ● Light
- ●● Medium
- ●●● Heavy

Chemicals called prostaglandins are released when menstruation begins. They cause your intestines and uterus to contract, leading to diarrhea and cramps. Medications such as ibuprofen and naproxen can help by decreasing the production of prostaglandins.

Record any symptoms you might have during your period, including cravings, your mood, cramps, aches, breast tenderness, and anything you did to feel better!

PMS Symptoms:

Day 1:

Day 2:

Day 3:

Day 4:

Day 5:

Day 6:

Day 7:

Notes:

_____ _____
         Month   Year

		1	2	3	4	5
6	7	8	9	10	11	12
13	14	15	16	17	18	19
20	21	22	23	24	25	26
27	28	29	30	31		

Days Since Last Period: ☐

Count the number of days in between the first day of each cycle, then take the average of several cycles to find out long your cycles are!

Key

● Light
●● Medium
●●● Heavy

Oral contraceptives are a great option for regulating periods. They can also help control heavy periods and decrease acne. Ask your doctor if they could be right for you.

Record any symptoms you might have during your period, including cravings, your mood, cramps, aches, breast tenderness, and anything you did to feel better!

PMS Symptoms:

Day 1:

Day 2:

Day 3:

Day 4:

Day 5:

Day 6:

Day 7:

Notes:

_____ _____
          Month   Year

		1	2	3	4	5
6	7	8	9	10	11	12
13	14	15	16	17	18	19
20	21	22	23	24	25	26
27	28	29	30	31		

Days Since Last Period: ☐

Count the number of days in between the first day of each cycle, then take the average of several cycles to find out long your cycles are!

Key

- ● Light
- ●● Medium
- ●●● Heavy

Cravings? Protein helps stabilize blood sugar and increase feelings of fullness after a meal. Including plenty of protein rich foods in your diet can help control cravings. High protein foods include eggs, nuts, dairy, seafood, and meat.

Record any symptoms you might have during your period, including cravings, your mood, cramps, aches, breast tenderness, and anything you did to feel better!

PMS Symptoms:

Day 1:

Day 2:

Day 3:

Day 4:

Day 5:

Day 6:

Day 7:

Notes:

_____ _____
       Month   Year

		1	2	3	4	5
6	7	8	9	10	11	12
13	14	15	16	17	18	19
20	21	22	23	24	25	26
27	28	29	30	31		

Days Since Last Period: ☐

Count the number of days in between the first day of each cycle, then take the average of several cycles to find out long your cycles are!

Key
- ● Light
- ●● Medium
- ●●● Heavy

PMS? Research has shown that women with higher intakes of calcium and vitamin D are less likely to develop PMS. Calcium from food is better absorbed than calcium from supplements. Calcium rich foods include milk, cheese, yogurt, fortified orange juice or soymilk. Leafy greens are also a great source of calcium!

Record any symptoms you might have during your period, including cravings, your mood, cramps, aches, breast tenderness, and anything you did to feel better!

PMS Symptoms:

Day 1:

Day 2:

Day 3:

Day 4:

Day 5:

Day 6:

Day 7:

Notes:

Month _____ Year _____

		1	2	3	4	5
6	7	8	9	10	11	12
13	14	15	16	17	18	19
20	21	22	23	24	25	26
27	28	29	30	31		

Days Since Last Period: ☐

Count the number of days in between the first day of each cycle, then take the average of several cycles to find out long your cycles are!

Key

- 💧 Light
- 💧💧 Medium
- 💧💧💧 Heavy

Stress can contribute to how intense PMS symptoms are. Take a few minutes out of your day to relax and take a deep breath. There are lots of great resources online on meditation.

Record any symptoms you might have during your period, including cravings, your mood, cramps, aches, breast tenderness, and anything you did to feel better!

PMS Symptoms:

Day 1:

Day 2:

Day 3:

Day 4:

Day 5:

Day 6:

Day 7:

Notes:

_____ _____
　　　　　　　　　　　Month　　　　　　　　　Year

		1	2	3	4	5
6	7	8	9	10	11	12
13	14	15	16	17	18	19
20	21	22	23	24	25	26
27	28	29	30	31		

Days Since Last Period: ☐

Count the number of days in between the first day of each cycle, then take the average of several cycles to find out long your cycles are!

Key

- 💧 Light
- 💧💧 Medium
- 💧💧💧 Heavy

In addition to causing cancer and wrinkles, a recent study has shown that smoking, especially in early adulthood, may increase a woman's risk for PMS symptoms.

Record any symptoms you might have during your period, including cravings, your mood, cramps, aches, breast tenderness, and anything you did to feel better!

PMS Symptoms:

Day 1:

Day 2:

Day 3:

Day 4:

Day 5:

Day 6:

Day 7:

Notes:

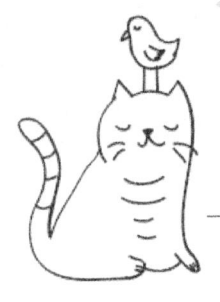

_____ _____
Month   Year

		1	2	3	4	5
6	7	8	9	10	11	12
13	14	15	16	17	18	19
20	21	22	23	24	25	26
27	28	29	30	31		

Days Since Last Period: ☐

Count the number of days in between the first day of each cycle, then take the average of several cycles to find out long your cycles are!

Key
- ● Light
- ●● Medium
- ●●● Heavy

Bloated? It doesn't sound intuitive, but drinking plenty of water can help with bloating. The water helps flush out extra sodium from your body, reducing water retention. How much water did you drink today?

Record any symptoms you might have during your period, including cravings, your mood, cramps, aches, breast tenderness, and anything you did to feel better!

PMS Symptoms:

Day 1:

Day 2:

Day 3:

Day 4:

Day 5:

Day 6:

Day 7:

Notes:

_____ _____
           Month   Year

		1	2	3	4	5
6	7	8	9	10	11	12
13	14	15	16	17	18	19
20	21	22	23	24	25	26
27	28	29	30	31		

Days Since Last Period: ☐

Count the number of days in between the first day of each cycle, then take the average of several cycles to find out long your cycles are!

Key
- ♦ Light
- ♦♦ Medium
- ♦♦♦ Heavy

Fatigued? PMS can cause you to feel extra tired compared to usual. It is important to have an established sleeping schedule and sleep on time every night. Aim for around 7 to 8 hours of beauty sleep each day.

Record any symptoms you might have during your period, including cravings, your mood, cramps, aches, breast tenderness, and anything you did to feel better!

PMS Symptoms:

Day 1:

Day 2:

Day 3:

Day 4:

Day 5:

Day 6:

Day 7:

Notes:

_____
Month   Year

		1	2	3	4	5
6	7	8	9	10	11	12
13	14	15	16	17	18	19
20	21	22	23	24	25	26
27	28	29	30	31		

Days Since Last Period: ☐

Count the number of days in between the first day of each cycle, then take the average of several cycles to find out long your cycles are!

Key

- ● Light
- ●● Medium
- ●●● Heavy

Being on your period may make you feel gross. But remember, your vagina is like a self-cleaning oven. You do not need to put anything inside to clean it. This includes douches, which can lead to vaginal infections.

Record any symptoms you might have during your period, including cravings, your mood, cramps, aches, breast tenderness, and anything you did to feel better!

PMS Symptoms:

Day 1:

Day 2:

Day 3:

Day 4:

Day 5:

Day 6:

Day 7:

Notes:

_____ Month _____ Year _____

		1	2	3	4	5
6	7	8	9	10	11	12
13	14	15	16	17	18	19
20	21	22	23	24	25	26
27	28	29	30	31		

Days Since Last Period: ☐

Count the number of days in between the first day of each cycle, then take the average of several cycles to find out long your cycles are!

Key
- ● Light
- ●● Medium
- ●●● Heavy

Menstrual stains on your clothes? Soaking the item of clothing in cold water immediately can keep the blood from setting into the fabric. Follow with laundry soap as usual. For stubborn stains, hydrogen peroxide can help remove them. Just remember to spot test an inconspicuous area first.

Record any symptoms you might have during your period, including cravings, your mood, cramps, aches, breast tenderness, and anything you did to feel better!

PMS Symptoms:

Day 1:

Day 2:

Day 3:

Day 4:

Day 5:

Day 6:

Day 7:

Notes:

Month　　　_Year_

		1	2	3	4	5
6	7	8	9	10	11	12
13	14	15	16	17	18	19
20	21	22	23	24	25	26
27	28	29	30	31		

Days Since Last Period: ☐

Count the number of days in between the first day of each cycle, then take the average of several cycles to find out how long your cycles are!

Key
- 💧 Light
- 💧💧 Medium
- 💧💧💧 Heavy

Cramps? A natural way to help alleviate menstrual cramp pain is self massage. Massaging your lower abdomen (gently!) can encourage blood flow and relax the tense muscles. While you're at it, massage your lower back to help with any back pain.

Record any symptoms you might have during your period, including cravings, your mood, cramps, aches, breast tenderness, and anything you did to feel better!

PMS Symptoms:

Day 1:

Day 2:

Day 3:

Day 4:

Day 5:

Day 6:

Day 7:

Notes:

Year End Summary:
Cycle Lengths

Month 1	
Month 2	
Month 3	
Month 4	
Month 5	
Month 6	
Month 7	
Month 8	
Month 9	
Month 10	
Month 11	
Month 12	

Average Cycle Length: _____

Made in the USA
Coppell, TX
11 January 2022